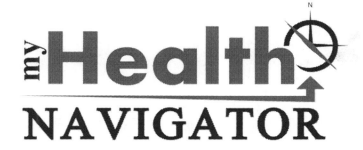

my Health NAVIGATOR

THE ROAD TO CHANGE

Dr. Michael A. Prytula ND

Contributors

Dr Mary Magnotta HBSc., MSc., ND

Dr Mike Um HBSc., ND

Acknowledgments

We would like to thank Diana Taylor, Joanna Barnett B.A., Meghan McNaughton HBSc., Kristin Oakley BHSc., Rayan Mokbel BHSc., MaryAnn Magnotta RN BA CNCC (C), and Silvia Magnotta BA RMT SIT for their support, patience and persistence in providing us with insightful feedback to manifest this book.

Table of Contents

**Please see the accompanying HealthNowHere video
at www.NaturoMedic.com**

LOOKING FOR A MIRACLE?

In many ways, we are all looking and waiting for a miracle, whether it is a health miracle, financial miracle, relationship miracle, etc. Who would not love the freedom of winning the lottery? But what exactly is a miracle? According to the Merriam-Webster dictionary, a miracle is an extraordinary event manifesting divine intervention in human affairs.

In a miracle, the responsibility lies on another party. In other words, there is nothing required of us and the miracle is provided by something/someone else. As appreciative as many of us would be of a miracle, what truly is the extent of our benefit and how much have we really learned? For instance, statistics have shown that lottery recipients of $50,000 to $150,000 are more likely to file for bankruptcy in the three to five years following their win. They chose not to take responsibility, not to change their habits and not to pay off their debt, therefore, they failed to learn from their experience.

Similar parallels may be drawn for recipients of healing miracles. Consider the man who, when given a second chance with an artificial/new heart, was met in the recovery room with a hot dog and a beer before being subsequently wheeled outside for a cigarette. It is difficult to question whether this person was particularly appreciative of their miracle. It is evident that they did not change the behavior that led to their current circumstance. It is well-known that the survival rate of people who have successfully quit smoking following coronary bypass surgery improves significantly compared to smokers that did not quit. Only 39% of smoker's bypass grafts are disease-free after 5 years as opposed to 52% of non-smokers. Self-improvement is essential to the long-term benefits of your miracle. These statistics beg the question of **whether we need a miracle to change our lives or can we initiate changes independently of divine intervention?**

The histories of medicine and miracles are closely interwoven. Jacalyn Duffin MD in her book, Medical Miracles, examined Vatican sources on 1,400 documented miracles from six continents and spanning four centuries. The majority of miracles were evidenced by medical care and physician testimony. Miracles remained while deaths continued suggesting God blessed a few with a healing miracle.

While many may continue to wait for their "miracle cure" or "miracle drug", you can begin shifting your understanding of health and the paradigm of a miracle. You can be blessed with good health! So what is the difference between a miracle cure and being blessed with good health? **A strategy, will power and a willingness to change are the three tools you need to begin making a difference in your future. A miracle is usually a one shot deal; however, the blessings of good health are infinite**.

The Chinese proverb "Give a man a fish and you feed him for a day. Teach a man to fish and you feed him for a lifetime" is a good example of being blessed with good health. By providing knowledge of a new skill, the man is now able to provide for himself and his family long-term and therefore is not always relying on another party to do the work. Knowledge is empowerment. Understanding the responsibility you have for your life and your health will make a difference on your road to success.

Are you ready to be blessed with good health?

YOUR HEALTH STRATEGY

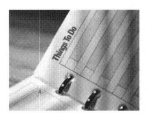

Empowerment begins with you. The road through life is a winding path, filled with ups, downs, curves and twists. Multiple challenges and potholes will threaten your way. Having a road map to navigate the most direct route is essential.

The road through life is unmistakably dependent upon your health. The strength and vigor of the mind, body and spirit are essential components that demand attention. Similar to car maintenance and regular oil changes, self-care is a priority that allows you to run optimally to face the obstacles ahead. Do not wait for your body to make a "noise" or start "leaking" before you get it serviced; take care of your health now. In the long-term, you cannot trade yourself in or buy a new model.

The Health Navigator is the road map designed to help you reach your health destination. It exposes the many potholes and obstacles you may encounter throughout your journey. The tools of the Navigator will teach you to conquer the challenges of health on your road through life. Assessing your health status is the first step on your path to success.

What are your health goals?

Has anyone ever asked you what your **health goals** are? If they did, what would you say?

I would like:

- more energy
- improved sleep
- live pain free
- exercise more
- eat healthier
- better digestion
- live longer
- female wellness
- allergy free
- be disease free
- increased clarity of thought
- no pharmaceuticals

Goals are a powerful and critical tool in your health journey. They keep you on course, provide direction and facilitate focus. Setting goals provides each of us with a personal challenge and enforces health-conscience behaviours.

The human brain is not only designed to function in a goal oriented pattern it actually thirsts for the power of objectives. An estimated 10% of the brain's full capacity is consciously employed on a regular basis. The remaining 90% is subconscious and goals have the ability to harness this latent potential.

Chemicals, known as neurotransmitters, perform daily tasks within the brain. Dopamine is released when goals are set, acting as a motivator and rewarding us when we achieve the desired outcome. The neurotransmitter helps control pleasure centers in the brain, encouraging a repeat of rewarding behaviours (habits). Having a healthy goal (a successful habit) is a great objective to become addicted to.

The potential of the brain to aid in maintaining goals is a crucial asset. The billion bits of information the brain constantly receives every second is selectively filtered. The Reticular Activating System (RAS) is the area of the brain responsible for this process. It decides what to accept or reject. When goals are set the RAS becomes activated to notice opportunities that will help in achieving your endeavor.

Taking care of you is a necessity. Writing down concrete goals is the first step to develop successful

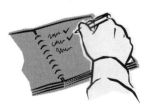

habits. Your physical, mental and spiritual state is begging for a commitment...it is time to set your starting point. There is a cost to not taking action.

What are you currently doing & how is that working for you?

Are you happy with your health? Are you getting results? Evaluating your current situation is an essential part of setting goals. Ask yourself what it is you really want to achieve:

- **Disease treatment ?**
- **Symptomatic relief ?**
- **Disease prevention ?**
- **Health optimization ?**

The importance of the outcome is one of the key factors facilitating your commitment to your goals.

A study by Gail Matthews from the Dominican University revealed some interesting conclusions about the benefits of setting goals. Matthews assigned volunteers from a broad range of ages and backgrounds to five different groups. Each group was asked to determine goals for a four-week time period; some were to just think about them; some were to write their goals down and others were asked to write progress reports to a friend as they completed their goals. The group that was asked to write down their goals had 50% more success in completing them than those who were only asked to think about their goals. The group that was asked to be accountable to a friend for completing their goals saw the highest level of success by fulfilling 76% of their stated goals. These conclusions suggest that **writing out goals and being accountable** to keep them are a great way to achieve the things we want to do. For goals to be effective, feedback that reveals progress is a key component to your strategy.

Time will always be critical to long term success. Staying on track, finding availability and remaining motivated with your busy schedule are constant challenges. Learning to prioritize is also important. The brain will routinely filter out goal-irrelevant activities, so set specific goals to enhance your performance. Discovering the appropriate strategy is critical to achieving complex objectives.

"The greatest danger for most of us is not that our aim is too high and we miss it, but that it is too low and we reach it." -
Michelangelo

What is your Health Strategy?

Has anyone ever asked you if you have a health strategy? Some of us have detailed strategies in place for how we plan to achieve success in our careers, security in our financial position or comfort in our retirement years. But how many of us have really thought about the need to create a personal **health strategy** that will allow us to enjoy all of these other achievements?

For most of us, our health strategy is a reactive one. We do not think about our health until something goes wrong. We can happily go for months or even years without seeing a health professional until an ache or pain warns us that something is not quite right. At that point, we schedule an appointment with our general practitioner (medical doctor). He/she does some blood work or possibly takes an x-ray or ultrasound of the problem area. After reviewing the results and doing other investigations, the practitioner makes a diagnosis and sends us on our way, possibly with some medication to treat the issue. We leave with the hope that it will be months or years before we need to see the doctor again.

Is this really a successful health strategy? Our bodies (and their proper functioning physically, mentally, and emotionally) are essential for everything that we do. We all have friends or relatives who have experienced life-altering challenges. They have been forever changed by the limitations placed on their body or mind by an illness. Do we place enough importance on the maintenance of our health? Are we willing to go the extra mile to do all that we can to ensure a healthy retirement, rather than have our poor health retire us?

Well-being should be a priority along with material growth. For the past three decades, the small Asian country of Bhutan has championed a new approach to development, which measures prosperity through GNH (Gross National Happiness) and the spiritual, physical, social and environmental health of its citizens rather than by the GDP (Gross Domestic Product) prosperity model. This approach is attracting a lot of interest.

It is NaturoMedic.com's desire to see a similar shift in our health care systems. Health can be a very controversial topic for a country or government. It is likely that elections have been lost or won over the subject of health care. Emphasis on a long-term health strategy by our mainstream medical system has been inconsistent at best and where the emphasis is put can make a world of difference...

Health**No**Where

Health**Now**Here!

NATUROMEDIC.COM'S HEALTH STRATEGY

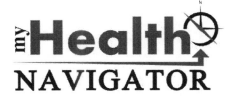

My Health Navigator is a tool designed to inform and encourage readers about an effective health strategy that has been successfully implemented with thousands of patients over the past twenty years. As doctors, authors and as a clinic, our purpose is to direct and walk alongside our patients and readers as they seek to reach their health goals. Our strategy is designed to address the true nature of disease and promote an attainable definition of health.

The World Health Organization (WHO) has defined health as "a state of complete physical, mental and social well-being and not merely the absence of disease or infirmity." Despite no amendments to this statement since 1948, mainstream medicine continues to define health as the absence of disease. Like the WHO, NaturoMedic.com seeks not only to view health as the absence of disease, but also as a state of well-being in which disease causing factors are identified and addressed in every area of an individual's life. By striving for continual physical, emotional, spiritual and social optimization, we at NaturoMedic.com aspire to increase vitality to **Give Life to the Living™!**

Our strategy is to identify where you are on **The Health Continuum™ in order to treat disease, treat functional disorders and prevent disease while progressing towards health optimization**. In order to accomplish this, health improvements are made through successive therapeutic sessions, increasing **quality of life, vitality and energy**. There are many disease causing factors that require identification and isolation in order to attain and maintain optimal well-being. At NaturoMedic.com, our health strategy includes 5 key principles.

The Health Continuum™:
Functional Disorder vs. Pathological Disease

The first foundational principle in our strategy is The Health Continuum™, which illustrates the progression of disease. A visit to your medical doctor (MD) will usually begin with a symptom. In some cases, the MD may run multiple tests that do not present a diagnosis; their investigations come back within normal limits. There may be no signs of a pathological disease, but you still do not feel well. This may actually be due to a functional problem.

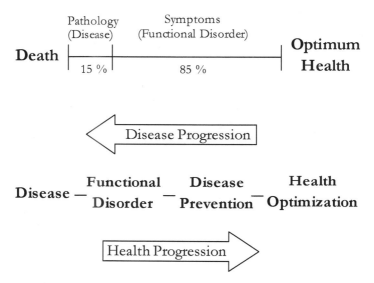

In fact, **85% of visits to MDs are for functional problems and not pathological ones.** A functional disorder requires a tune up rather than significant intervention by your MD. In other words, you are not sick enough to qualify for treatment under the current system of healthcare. Therefore, you are left with symptoms but without a long-term strategy to successfully address them. Interestingly, Traditional Chinese Medicine functioned completely opposite to our system today. **In ancient times, Chinese doctors were only paid as they maintained the health of their patients. If the patient became ill, the doctor was expected to provide free treatment. Their main goal was to promote**

14

optimal health and rectify functional disorders before pathology became established. As NDs our focus is ultimately to guide you through the Health Continuum™ by providing disease treatment, functional disorder treatment and disease prevention on the road to achieving optimal health.

The Health Cup Analogy™:
Multifactorial vs. Monocausal

Another distinctive principle of our health strategy is that at NaturoMedic.com, we always look for the root cause of the problem. What are the factors causing poor health? There are usually several in a chronic condition (multifactorial) or there may be just one in an acute condition like an injury (monocasual). Modern pharmaceutical medicine prefers the monocausal disease philosophy as this promotes the idea of the magic bullet or miracle pill; one pill to address one symptom, or one intervention to address one symptom. The Health Navigator proposes a different strategy. All possible factors are taken into consideration in order to properly assess and treat the cause of your health concerns. Humans are complicated beings. Over 1 trillion chemical reactions occur in our bodies every second. Neurons fire every millisecond. We are very complex organisms indeed.

The Health Cup Analogy™: Imagine your body as a cup which represents your well-being. Your health cup is constantly being filled by various factors (these could include: pollution, diet, stress, microorganisms, etc.). Overall these burdens can be categorized into 5 main sections: Environment, Lifestyle, Body, Mind and Spirit (Figure 1).

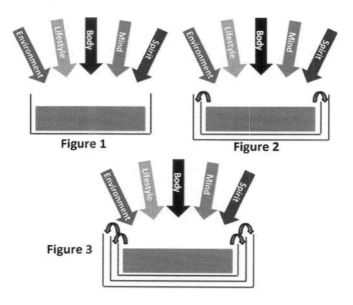

Multiple factors accumulate as we progress through life and eventually your cup overflows resulting in functional symptoms or possibly disease. Most prescription medications regrettably do not address the causal problems. Instead they give you a larger cup to catch the overflow (Figure 2). **The symptoms are given temporary relief,** (the magic bullet or miracle drug) **but the factors causing those symptoms are not eliminated, so the cup overflows again. This necessitates another stronger prescription** (another miracle drug) **to deal with an ever–expanding litany of symptoms, but does not address the multitude of causes** (Figure 3). In order to obtain long-term health, we must treat the cause by identifying, isolating and/or altering the factors filling up your cup. Emptying your cup of these negative influences will lead to a true recovery rather than a suppression of symptoms.

Pharmaceutical treatment of headaches is an excellent example of an immediate Band-Aid solution. Tylenol provides a bigger cup (Figure 2), however, it does not isolate any factors actually causing the headache. If causal factors, like diet, stress and environment are ignored, then after a while, the Tylenol fails to work, requiring stronger medication. This creates a larger cup, but none of the causal factors have been treated. The cycle continues as the medications progress to Imitrex, then Cafergot, Fiorinal, nerve blocks or botox (Figure 3). These provide symptomatic relief, but the cause is still not addressed. Arthritis and heart disease are conditions which follow similar patterns.

- For arthritis, pain relief begins with Tylenol or Advil, followed by Non-Steroidal Anti-Inflammatories (Celebrex, Naproxen), then steroids, onto chemotherapeutic medications such as Methotrexate and eventually joint replacement.
- For heart disease, various blood pressure medications are prescribed, followed by blood thinners and cholesterol lowering pills. Gradually, the number of prescriptions for each of the above are increased while the patient is being continuously monitored for when to provide surgical intervention.

More prescriptions provide a larger cup, yet no one is isolating the factors filling up the cup and contributing to these disease conditions. Discovering the various causal factors is essential to eliminating disease and reaching your health goals.

Environment

- Air Quality
- Environmental Allergies
- Water Quality
- Chemicals & Solvents
- Pesticides
- Heavy Metals
- Vaccines
- Microorganisms
- Weather
- Radiation & Electromagnetic Fields

Lifestyle

- Alcohol
- Coffee
- Blood Sugar
- Pop
- Smoking
- Street Drugs
- Diet & Food Allergies
- Vitamin & Mineral Deficiencies
- Hygiene
- Exercise
- Prescription Drugs
- Water Quantity
- Obesity & Body Mass Index

Body

- Circulation & Blood Pressure
- Genetics
- Hormones
- Structural Damage
- Weak & Diseased Organs

Mind

- Sleep
- Social Network
- Stress Management
- Finances
- Joy/No Joy
- Anxiety/Worry
- Fear/Fright
- Grief
- Anger
- Depression
- Work
- Sex
- Our Subconscious

Spirit

- Belief: Faith & Hope
- Forgiveness
- Love
- Spiritual Doors

Everyone is physiologically unique and the roadmap to health is dependent upon assessing the whole person. Modern medicine has isolated the body into different segments, (i.e. dermatology, endocrinology, rheumatology, etc.) with each specialization acting independently of the other. At NaturoMedic.com, we acknowledge the complex interrelationships of environment, lifestyle, body, mind and spirit, thus believing each segment works synergistically with the others. The person as a whole must be taken into account in order to create an effective plan to continue in the right direction on The Health Continuum™.

Healing Crisis vs. Disease Crisis

The third foundational principle in our health strategy is the well accepted naturopathic concept of a healing crisis. The path to health is not easy; you may feel temporarily worse before you feel better. These may not be the encouraging words you wish to read, although the change of symptoms is usually a positive sign. A healing crisis is associated with the emptying of your cup and removal of a disease causing factor. When the burden is isolated some symptoms initially become worse as the body now has more energy to focus on healing another area. This is what is commonly known as a **healing crisis**. Your energy and symptoms are the keys to determining whether this is a healing crisis or a disease crisis. According to Constantine Hering, the father of American homeopathy, as healing progresses, symptoms appear in the reverse order of occurrence, from the top down, inside out and from the most vital to least vital organs. Therefore, if your energy is increasing while symptoms worsen or old ailments return, you are going through a healing crisis. In contrast, a **disease crisis** is when the overall progression of symptoms, energy and disease continue to deteriorate. The experience of a healing crisis, while not initially enjoyable, can often be accompanied by a sensation of euphoria as the burden in the cup is being eliminated. Do not let the initial stages of a healing crisis discourage you. Stay focused and remember your ultimate goal.

The Weakest Link™

The fourth of our five health strategy principles is the importance of supporting The Weakest Link™. To reiterate, at NaturoMedic.com we acknowledge the complex interrelationships of the environment, lifestyle, body, mind and spirit. The various physiological functions and processes of your body can be represented by an intricate chain. Each link represents a different organ, hormone, muscle, neurotransmitter, enzyme, protein, etc. The strength of the chain is dependent upon the connection of each link. In regards to health, the common expression "a chain is only as strong as its weakest link" holds true.

When one area is not functioning properly, the body attempts to compensate for the weakness. At NaturoMedic.com, we begin the health journey by systematically isolating disease causing factors and supporting the most fragile link to help rebuild your system. By strengthening The Weakest Link™, the whole chain becomes stronger, resolving many symptoms without the need for further intervention. The body has the ability to heal itself if given the right conditions and support. *Vis medicatrix naturae* is the latin phrase that refers to the healing power of nature. It is one of the founding beliefs of Naturopathic Medicine. It is our essential life energy (*Qi*, vital force) that helps us to heal and maintain balance. By identifying obstacles and reinforcing areas of weakness, we are fostering the power of the *vis* to promote healing as your cup is purged. There are many layers to health. On your journey, each layer must be successfully peeled away, like an onion, to reach your optimal health.

Docere (Doctor as Teacher)

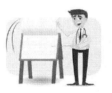

The final key principle of NaturoMedic.com's health strategy is the naturopathic concept of doctor as teacher. Education is critical to treating disease and progressing toward the achievement of optimal health. A Naturopathic Doctor (ND) plays a very crucial role in this process; an ND acts as a teacher. Disease can manifest in a variety of forms. By understanding the factors contributing to the problem and how they can be corrected, health is attained. The knowledge contained in the Health Navigator will empower and motivate you to make informed decisions and take control of your health.

What to Expect

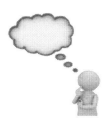

NaturoMedic.com's health strategy incorporates these 5 key principles as well as methods of accountability to ensure commitment and goal attainment. Obtaining a full health history is essential for identifying obstacles and individualizing your strategy. There are health practitioners whose strategy is to give supplements that address every issue at once. You will feel better, but unfortunately you will always be dependent upon the supplements or the practitioner to maintain your health. At NaturoMedic.com we take a systematic approach. By isolating factors in a sequential way and supporting The Weakest Link™, we can provide minimal supplementation, save you money and help you take control of your own health. The education about disease causing factors is invaluable to your success. When you learn how disease progresses, you can actively work towards disease prevention and the optimization of your health.

It is necessary to understand that your present state of health may be the result of an entire lifetime of habits. Therefore, to expect an overnight cure is unrealistic. Healing is a process that takes time and commitment.

The Road to Change

At NaturoMedic.com, we do not chase symptoms. We seek to find the root of the problem and address it. To achieve this we want to know all about you!

To assist you in getting the most out of your doctor visits and attaining your health goals, we have created tools to help you track your progress on a routine basis. The **Symptom Tracker™** and **Lab Tracker™** are designed to keep you in tune with your body, allowing you to see the long-term change in your health and motivating you to fulfill your health goals. The **Pill Minder™** is a great addition for maintaining your treatment schedule. Knowing when to administer medications and observing their effects on your symptoms can significantly amplify your progress. By utilizing these tools you will be able to monitor your health progress over time. This will boost your self-confidence and provide the impetus to push forward to your goal of disease prevention and health optimization. These tools are currently available in hard copy form at NaturoMedic.com.

At NaturoMedic.com our goal is to work with you to provide education, service and access to effective healing therapies geared towards giving you the health results you desire. In order to be successful, your cooperation as a member of your own health team is essential. All the necessary forms, tools and products are available, however, without your participation it will be difficult to achieve the results you desire. This is equivalent to asking us to wrestle a disease to the ground with one arm tied behind our backs.

Before entering into an effective treatment relationship, NaturoMedic.com will propose a **Health Commitment™**. The NaturoMedic.com team is determined to provide safe, effective, individualized treatment that addresses your concerns and is intended to provide disease prevention while working towards optimal health. NaturoMedic.com will strive to reach these goals throughout your treatment program and we encourage your participation by giving us your feedback.

The opportunity of having a guide with an effective strategy for achieving your goals will accelerate your journey to health.

MODERN MEDICINE:
THE CURRENT LEGACY

The success of modern medicine in achieving health is frequently assessed by measuring life expectancy and death rates. The discovery of the miracle drug, penicillin, in 1941, contributed to the largest increase in life expectancy. In the following decade, the average life span in the U.S. moved from 62.9 years of age to 68.2 (+5.3 years). Through pharmaceutical development, modern medicine has succeeded in achieving longevity, however the quality of longevity needs to be assessed. **We are living longer but are we living well? Over the past half-century, the death rates of all diseases (with the exception of heart disease and stroke) have either plateaued or increased in both Canada and the United States.** This evidence illustrates that modern medicine's health strategy is not having significant success at addressing the major causes of illness (See Figure 4 & 5).

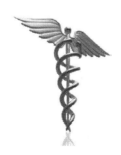

Age-adjusted death rates for selected leading causes of death: United States, 1958-2010

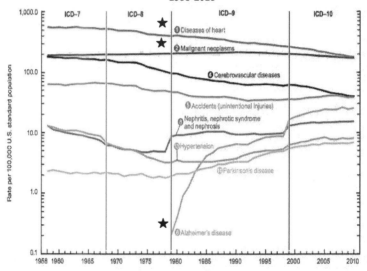

Figure 4. Age-adjusted leading causes of death in the United States from 1958-2010. The death rates of heart disease, cancer and Alzheimer's disease are highlighted, showing little to no change in cancer rates (malignant neoplasms), some decrease in heart disease and an exponential increase in Alzheimer's disease. Source:http://www.cdc.gov/nchs/data/nvsr/nvsr61/nvsr 61_04.pdf

Heart Disease and Stroke (Cerebrovascular Disease)

According to Health Canada, smoking is related to 29% of deaths caused by heart disease and stroke. From 1965-2011, the number of 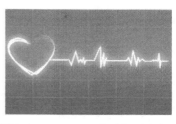 smokers declined by 64.5% in men and 60.5% in women. **The change in heart and stroke deaths over the past decades can therefore be directly linked to the reduction in smoking**. In fact, within 20 minutes of quitting smoking, blood pressure and heart rate return to normal. Within 2 weeks, circulation and lung function improve. Within a year, the risk of heart disease is reduced by half. Finally, after 15 years of living smoke-free, heart disease risks are the same as that of non-smokers. The health benefits associated with quitting smoking directly correlates with the visible decrease in cardiovascular deaths related to smoking. Smoking is only one factor that contributes to deaths caused by heart disease and stroke. Other factors include: infection, heavy metals, nitric oxide deficiency and inflammation.

Cancer (Malignant Neoplasms)

In the past 50 years, cancer death rates have not changed significantly. Any marginal improvement in cancer incidence is thought to be due to the decline in smoking.

Both the Canadian and American Lung Associations confirm that it takes at least 10 years after quitting smoking for lung cancer risks to be decreased by half. **In tobacco smoke there are more than 7,000 chemicals and at least 69 of which are known carcinogens.** Inhalation of heavy metals found in tobacco and cigarette smoke, including arsenic, cadmium, chromium, nickel and lead, also contribute to various forms of cancer. Particularly oral (mouth, throat, esophagus, larynx), bladder, lung and pancreatic cancers. With fewer people smoking, exposure to these chemicals and carcinogens has been greatly reduced. Therefore, cancer rates should have declined significantly.

Lung cancer rates in men improved two decades after smoking decreased by 20%. **If we factor in the declining number of people exposed to smoking's toxic burden, cancer in general has actually increased significantly.** With few exceptions, the incidence of most types of cancer has actually metastasized or shown no change. Smoking is therefore not the only factor driving cancer.

Leading causes of death and percent change from 2000 to 2009, Canada			
Total population	30,685,730	33,628,571	+8.75
Cause of Mortality	Mortality 2000	Mortality 2009	Change (%)
All causes of death	218,062	238,418	+8.5
1	Cancer	62,672	71,125	+13.5
2	Heat disease	55,070	49,271	-10.5
3	Stroke	15,576	14,105	-9.4
4	Chronic lower respiratory disease	9,813	10,859	+9.6
5	Accidents (unintentional injury)	8,589	10,250	+16.2
6	Diabetes mellitus	6,714	6,923	+3.0
7	Alzheimer's disease	5,007	6,281	+25.4
8	Influenza and pneumonia	4,966	5,826	+14.8
9	Intentional self-harm	3,606	3,890	+7.3
10	Kidney disease	3,136	3,609	+13.1
	All other causes	42,913	56,279	+23.7

Figure 5. Changes in causes of death in Canada between 2000 and 2009. The death rates of cancer, heart disease, Alzheimer's disease, influenza and pneumonia exhibited the most change. Cancer and heart disease continue to be the leading causes of death. Interestingly, while cancer mortality rates have increased by +13.5%, death by heart disease has decreased by -10.5% over the 9 year span. Source:http://www.statcan.gc.ca/dailyquotidien/120725/t 120725b001-eng.htm.

In the past 50 years, much has been learned about the varying complexities of cancer. Cancer is not caused by one factor, it is caused by a multitude of factors. Therefore a multifaceted approach emphasizing a reduction in the known contributors to the formation and propagation of cancer would be an essential part of any successful strategy.

In 1971, President Nixon declared war on cancer. **It is evident that with cancer death rates as high as they are, the $105 billion invested by the American Cancer Institute since the war started, has not been successful at significantly decreasing mortality rates while preserving quality of life.** Canada is not doing any better, considering the increase in investments in cancer research in the past five years to as much as $545.5 million. In 2010 the National Cancer Institute (NCI) reported the annual cost for cancer care in the US was $125 billion dollars. NCI projected the 2020 costs would be $158-207 billion (in 2010 dollars).

Do we not deserve better results from our investment?

Alzheimer's Disease

Alzheimer's is now considered the most feared disease over any other life-threatening illness. In the U.S., **Alzheimer's deaths have increased approximately 130 fold (13,000%) in the last 30 years, as seen in Figure 4.** In 2010, over 35.6 million people worldwide were living with dementia. These exponentially rising rates have contributed to the mounting fear over one's future. **The inability to care for oneself is the primary concern that significantly minimizes one's hopes of living with dignity and ultimately dying with dignity**. To add to this increasing burden, as many as 15.5 million family and friends are currently providing around the clock care to loved ones suffering from Alzheimer's and dementia. This increased burden on loved one's lives (socially, financially and relationally) is the biggest worry among the aging population. Followed by the loss of the recollection of family and friends and life memories.

If this is longevity, then what is modern medicine's legacy?

Disability

In 2006, 14.3% of the population (4.4 million Canadians) reported being on disability. **Factoring for population growth, over five years from 2001-2006, an additional 1/4 million (250,000) working-age Canadians were registered as disabled.** In 2012, data showed that 1 in 10 (10%) of Canadians aged 15-64 (working-age) had a disability, compared to 1 in 3 (33%) among those aged 65 and older. American statistics were similar with 9.9% of the working-age population (aged 16 to 64) reported having a disability in 2012.

Unfortunately, the increase in disability rates does not stop there. Alarmingly, the ones most precious and defenseless in our society, our children, have also seen a dramatic rise in disability. **Half of all children aged 4 and under in Canada have reported at least one disability** in 2006, including asthma, severe allergies, ADD/ADHD and autism. In the U.S., the greatest rate of increase in childhood disability was seen throughout the 1990s, with **disability increasing 3 fold (300%) in 5 years from 300,000 in 1990 to 900,000 children in 1995.**

Pharmaceutical Drugs

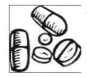 Are we suggesting that the current Canadian or American health care system should be discarded? Of course not. However, we do need to recognize the limitations of their strategy. When only the symptoms of a problem are addressed, a Band-Aid solution is provided and the root cause will never be cured. In North America, prescription drug trends have increased exponentially over the past 20 years. According to Statistics Canada, in 2005 alone, pharmacists dispensed **on average 35 prescriptions per person aged 60 to 79 and 74 prescriptions per person ages 80 or older, with an overall average of 14 prescriptions** for every Canadian citizen. In 2011, American doctors wrote 4.02 billion prescriptions, which if distributed equally, equates to about 13 prescriptions per citizen. Society today places a lot of value on quick fixes and instant results - expecting the same in the area of health. Unfortunately, modern medicines overuse of pharmaceuticals does not lend itself to long term strategies and results.

"He is the best physician that knows the worthlessness of most medicines." -Benjamin Franklin

Healthcare Expenditures

In the U.S., **from 1960 to 2008,** total annual national health care **expenditures increased from $28 billion to $2,339 billion** and total 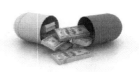 private health care costs have gone up from $21 billion to $1,232 billion. When looking at per capita expenses, **costs have nearly doubled in Canada and the U.S. between 1995 and 2007!**

Modern Medicine: Legacy Summary

While current life expectancy has increased over the past century, the data suggests that our mortality rates and quality of life have not improved, thus *HealthNoWhere.* Disability rates continue to rise in Canada and the U.S., along with poor returns in health outcomes from healthcare investments. Simply put, the current healthcare strategy is flawed. We need to explore a new approach. Consider if only 10% of current funding were granted to a truly successful health strategy! *HealthNowHere!*

Einstein's definition of Insanity: *"Doing the same thing over and over again and expecting different results."*

LESSONS FROM HISTORY

We need to be willing to invest in a health strategy that will target the root causes of our health concerns and commit to making the changes necessary to achieve our health goals. Similar 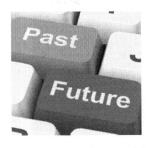 health strategies have existed throughout the world. For instance, **Traditional Chinese Medicine has continued to emphasize long-term health for over 5000 years.** Homeopathy has existed for the past 200 years and has stressed the importance of disease prevention and treating the underlying disease causing factors. **In North America, the first homeopathic hospital was opened in 1832. By the early 1900s, there were 22 homeopathic medical schools, 100 homeopathic hospitals and over 1,000 homeopathic pharmacies in the United States. Mortality (death) rates in homeopathic hospitals were often 50% to 88% less than those in medical hospitals.** This well-established profession is commonly practiced, most notably in India. These two methods of medicine are examples that a health care system designed to conquer the root cause and prevent disease can exist.

Moreover, it further demonstrates that this type of health strategy, which at one time was established in North America, has the potential for resurgence in our current medical system. NaturoMedic.com approaches health from this angle. Our hope is that more and more people will come to recognize the need for greater continuity in our health care system. Instead of tearing down the existing health care structure, it is our aim to see it improved as we build on the many things it already has to offer. Our desire is to see our patients taking steps to achieve optimal health in every area of their life. Establishing what you would like to achieve, setting high goals, embracing a proven strategy and developing methods of accountability are indispensable to obtaining concrete results. You can now begin being blessed with good health on your winding path through life.

--"Dream it. Plan it. Do it"--

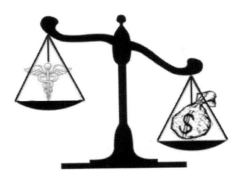

THE COST OF LONG TERM HEALTH

Visiting a Naturopathic Doctor (ND) for the first time often raises a few questions. What will the ND do? What will they prescribe? Will they use needles? What do I have to do? A primary concern of many is the cost. **What you may not know is that the cost of Naturopathic visits are covered under some company health insurance plans. Please check your plan to see exactly what you are eligible for.** A regular visit to a Medical Doctor is often for an acute condition that needs immediate attention, while your next visit may not be until a new concern arises. However, the treatment plan you receive from a

39

Naturopathic Doctor will be different than that of a Medical Doctor. Acute situations do arise from time to time, however, for Naturopathic Healthcare, regular visits are a part of our strategy to help you achieve health optimization and disease prevention. Ultimately, from an ND you will receive an individually customized treatment plan that addresses your acute and long-term concerns, giving you full control of your health care.

For many Canadians, unlike our American counterparts, this may be your first experience paying for health care, however, have you considered dental visits? Many benefit plans cover little to none of your treatment. We often do not give a second thought to the value of our trips to the dentist; we are paying for their knowledge, training, education and equipment to address long-term prevention of tooth decay or cosmetic beautification of our teeth. **Like Naturopathic Medicine, dentistry is just one example of health care not covered by Provincial Health Insurance (Canada) or Medicaid and Medicare (U.S.), but should your mouth receive more attention by equally educated professionals than the rest of your body?** There are many misconceptions in the education and training of Naturopathic Doctors as compared to Medical Doctors or Dentists, when in fact the length of time obtaining an education and cost of tuition are comparable (See Appendix).

In addition to the training of your ND, you are also paying for the knowledge, skills and judgment of the physician, and the experience at a professional facility.

As on the Health Continuum (p 13-15) you are paying for disease treatment, treatment of functional disorders, disease prevention and health optimization. Let us use the analogy of a car in place of your health. Acute situations, like a flat tire (a symptom), may have happened overnight and are quick to fix. A chronic condition on the other hand did not happen overnight, like a seized transmission where there were years of abuse and neglected service. With a chronic disease there is additional pathology, lab tests, treatment etc… more than what is needed for keeping the body and the immune system strong, this will therefore take longer to resolve after years of neglect. Like a car, your health needs to be maintained on a regular basis to prevent serious illness and increased medication costs. In order to keep your car running longer, it requires regular maintenance, oil changes, tune-ups etc… **To keep your car at peak performance (health optimization), regular maintenance (disease prevention) is required. If your car is neglected, it will eventually begin to** break down (functional symptoms), leading to costly mechanical repairs (disease treatment), such as rebuilding the engine, which could leave you paying up to $5000. A serious illness can be the equivalent of getting your engine rebuilt, as large-scale interventions are required as opposed to regular maintenance. There is a difference between maintenance and correction of an injury or disease. In maintaining one's appearance the average person spends about $75 for a haircut, $100 for colouring and $80 for a manicure and pedicure, not to mention the costs for cosmetic dental work (braces, whitening, etc.). These services are not covered by insurance, yet they are necessities that many are willing to pay for without question. Doesn't your health deserve just as much attention and room in your budget as beautification services or your car?

In 2014, the U.S. spent the largest amount on health care ($8,508/person), yet it has the lowest overall healthcare quality out of 11 industrialized nations. Canada spent $5,988/person, for its underperforming system, ranking 10th out of 11 for healthcare quality. Ultimately you cannot put a price tag on your health, but you want to be confident you are receiving the best and most comprehensive health care possible for the cost. If you wish to compare Alternative Health

Practitioners, please consider the following: knowledge, equipment, training, tools, experience, the professional facility and most importantly, that you are seeing an accredited Naturopathic Doctor. **Your healthcare is in your hands, so be sure to invest in a properly trained professional with a strategy that promotes disease treatment, symptomatic relief, while working towards health optimization and disease prevention.**

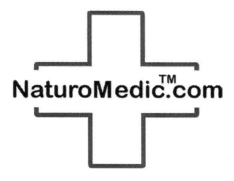

SUMMARY

My Health Navigator: The Road to Change is designed to expose the many potholes and obstacles impeding your journey to your health destination. Goal setting and an effective health strategy are mandatory for success in your endeavor. As the Navigator tools teach you how to conquer the challenges of health on your road through life, they also establish the benefit of accountability and commitment. At NaturoMedic.com, our integrated health strategy incorporates 5 key principles to expedite results and uphold persistence.

Thank you for taking the initial steps to learn about your health and work towards being blessed with good health.

We have empowered you with the knowledge you need to navigate the way through your journey of well-being. This strategy will remove the burdens of the Environment, Lifestyle, Body, Mind and Spirit to progress through The Health Continuum™ to health optimization. What you do with this wealth of knowledge is up to you; the ball is now in your court! With this in mind, we return to our original questions: **What are your health goals and what is your health strategy?**

Spread the **word** and be a leader of health. Your voyage will continue throughout life, but the story of your success will always be invaluable.

The NaturoMedic.com Team

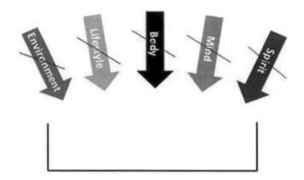

APPENDIX

The following charts demonstrate the equivalence in expenses and similar education, with medical doctors having more emphasis in surgery and pharmaceuticals in comparison to Naturopathic Doctors' pharmaceutical, nutritional and naturopathic interventions.

Canada, 2013/2014	Naturopathic Doctor (CCNM)	Medical Doctor	Dentist
Undergrad Degree (4 years @ 5,772/yr.)	$23,088	$23,088	$23,088
Post-graduate Tuition Cost per year	$20,600	*$12,438	*$17,324
Post-grad degree (4 years)	$82,400	$49,752	$69,296
Average Cost of Living (12,000-18,000 per year)	$96,000-$144,000	$96,000-$144,00	$96,000-$144,000
Average Cost of books, computers, equipment and incidentals	$22,000	$22,000	$22,000
Total:	$244,088-$292,088	$203,278-$251,278	$227,708-$275,708

*subsidized by the government.
Source:http://www.statcan.gc.ca/tables-tableaux/sum-som/l01/cst01/educ50a-eng.htm

When calculating the cost of one's education the income for the average person over 8 years should also be taken into consideration, as this income is lost during training. In the Greater Toronto Area, the average income over 8 years would equate to $208,000 and with a raise this amount could increase to about $250,000 ($26k/year). **With tuition, cost of living, books and supplies the average educational cost for an ND is actually closer to half a million dollars ($500,000). To incur this much debt, you require more than just dedication for 8 years, you need to have an unending passion for health and healing!**

ND vs. MD Education

	Naturopathic Medical School		Modern Medical School	
	NCNM	Bastyr	Yale	John Hopkins
Basic/Clinical Science	1548	1639	1420	1771
Allopathic Therapeutic & Counseling	2388	2068	2891 surgery	3391 surgery
Naturopathic Therapeutics	588	633	0	0
Therapeutic Nutrition	144	132	0	0
Total Hrs.:	4668	4472	4311	5280

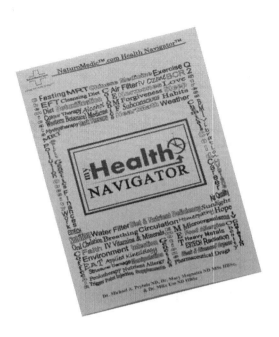

My Health Navigator is the next step on the road to health. This book is comprehensively created to identify the obstacles impeding your health. Each chapter focuses on a specific disease causing factor associated with the Environment, Lifestyle, Body, Mind and Spirit. My Health Navigator also includes explanations on specific treatments designed to support you, isolate the body burdening factors, optimize your health and prevent disease. Essentially it is your road map to success. This will undoubtedly provide answers and give direction to the path that is right for you. Pick up your copy to continue navigating your way to health.

To find a fully qualified Naturopathic Doctor in your area, consult the CAND in Canada (www.cand.ca) and the AANP (www.aanp.org) in the United States.

REFERENCES

1. http://www.merriam-webster.com/dictionary/miracle
2. Hoekstra, M. & Skiba, P.M. The Ticket to Easy Street? The Financial Consequences of Winning the Lottery Scott Hankins, University of Kentucky. Vanderbilt University Published on October 4, 2009
3. Voors AA, van Brussel BL, Plokker HW, et al. Smoking and cardiac events after venous coronary bypass surgery: a 15-year follow-up study. Circulation 1996; 93:42–7.
4. FitzGibbon GM, Leach AJ, Kafka HP. Atherosclerosis of coronary artery bypass grafts and smoking. CMAJ 1987;136:45
5. http://www.besancon-cardio.org/recommandations/cabg.pdf
6. International Thesaurus of Quotations, ed. Rhoda Thomas Tripp, p. 76, no. 3 (1970).
7. http://themedicalsanctuary.com.au/health/dopamine-and-reaching-our-goals/
8. http://michaelgholmes.com/why-goal-setters-change-the-world/
9. http://www.achieve-goal-setting-success.com/health-goals.html
10. http://toomuchonherplate.com/prioritize-yourself-and-be-more-effective-in-your-life
11. Locke, Edwin A.; Latham, Gary P. Building a practically useful theory of goal setting and task motivation: A 35-year odyssey. American Psychologist, Vol 57(9), Sep 2002, 705-717. http://faculty.washington.edu/janegf/goalsetting.html

12. Locke, Edwin A.; Shaw, Karyll N.; Saari, Lise M.; Latham, Gary P. Goal setting and task performance: 1969–1980.Psychological Bulletin, Vol 90(1), Jul 1981, 125-152.
http://www.dtic.mil/dtic/tr/fulltext/u2/a086584.pdf

13. http://www.guardian.co.uk/world/2012/dec/01/bhutan-wealth-happiness-counts

14. http://www.homeopathyworldcommunity.com/profiles/blogs/who-declares-homoeopathy-as

15. http://www.dominican.edu/dominicannews/study-backs-up-strategies-for-achieving-goals

16. http://www.who.int/about/definition/en/print.html

17. http://www.statcan.gc.ca/pub/82-003-x/2009001/article/10801/findings-resultats-eng.htm

18. http://www.naturalnews.com/037226_drug_prescriptions_medical_news_pills.html#ixzz2VLcPp7LD

19. Kroenke, K., & A.D.Mangelsdorff. Common Symptoms in Ambulatory Care: Incidence, Evaluation, Therapy & Outcome. American Journal of Medicine 86:262-266,   1989.
http://www.amjmed.com/article/0002-9343(89)90293-3/abstract

20. http://www.acupuncture.com/Conditions/pulse_prevent.htm

21. http://www.homeoint.org/biograph/heringen.htm

22. http://michaelhyatt.com/life-plan

23. http://michaelhyatt.com/the-power-of-incremental-change-over-time.html

24. Achor, Shawn; The Happiness Advantage, 2010. Pgs. 145-170.

25. Sanders, Tim. The Likeability Factor.

26. http://www.infoplease.com/ipa/A0005148.html

27. http://www.jameslefanu.com/books/the-rise-and-fall-of-modern-medicine-introduction
28. http://www.infoplease.com/ipa/A0005148.html
29. http://www.jameslefanu.com/books/the-rise-and-fall-of-modern-medicine-introduction
30. http://www.lung.org/stop-smoking/how-to-quit/why-quit/benefits-of-quitting/
31. http://www.lung.ca/protect-protegez/tobacco-tabagisme/quitting-cesser/benefits-bienfaits_e.ph
32. http://www.lung.org/stop-smoking/about-smoking/facts-figures/whats-in-a-cigarette.html
33. http://www.lung.org/stop-smoking/jow-to-quit/why-quit/benefits-of-quitting/
34. http://www.lung.ca/protect-protegez/tobacco-tabagisme/quitting-cesser/benefits-bienfaits_e.ph
35. http://www.lung.org/stop-smoking/about-smoking/facts-figures/whats-in-a-cigarette.html
36. http://www.scpr.org/news/2012/11/14/34931/do-you-fear-alzheimers-many-americans-do-poll-says/
37. http://www.cdc.gov/nchs/data/nvsr/nvsr61/nvsr61_04.pdf
38. http://www.heartandstroke.com/site/c.ikIQLcMWJtE/b.3483991/k.34A8/Statistics.htm
39. http://www.nytimes.com/2009/06/28/health/research/28cancer.html?pagewanted=all&_r=0
40. http://www.tobaccoreport.ca/2013/TobaccoUseinCanada_2013.pdf
41. http://www.statcan.gc.ca/daily-quotidien/120725/t120725b001-eng.htm
42. Int J Environ Res Public Health. 2013 Dec 20;11(1):202-17. doi: 10.3390/ijerph110100202. Toxic

metal concentrations in cigarettes obtained from U.S. smokers in 2009: results from the International Tobacco Control (ITC) United States survey cohort. (http://ezproxy.ccnm.edu:2077/pubmed/24452255) Caruso RV[1], O'Connor RJ[2], Stephens WE[3], Cummings KM[4], Fong GT[5]

43. The Scientific World Journal, Volume 2012 (2012), Article ID 729430, 5 pages, http://dx.doi.org/10.1100/2012/729430 Levels of Heavy Metals in Popular Cigarette Brands and Exposure to These Metals via Smoking, Muhammad Waqar Ashraf (http://www.hindawi.com/journals/tswj/2012/729430/)

44. O. Emre, H. Demir, E. Dogan, R. Esen, T. Gur, C. Demir, E. Gonullu, N. Turan and M. Özbay, "Plasma Concentrations of Some Trace Element and Heavy Metals in Patients with Metastatic Colon Cancer," *Journal of Cancer Therapy*, Vol. 4 No. 6, 2013, pp. 1085-1090. doi: 10.4236/jct.2013.46124. (http://www.scirp.org/journal/PaperInformation.aspx?PaperID=34987#.U48rWcfgW5N)

45. Pancreatic cancer clusters and arsenic-contaminated drinking water wells in Florida Wen Liu-Mares, Jill A MacKinnon, Recinda Sherman, Lora E Fleming, Caio Rocha-Lima, Jennifer J Hu, David J Lee BMC Cancer March 2013, 13:111 (http://link.springer.com/article/10.1186/1471-2407-13-111)

46. Is Cadmium a Cause of Human Pancreatic Cancer? Gary G. Schwartz, Isildinha M. Reis (http://cebp.aacrjournals.org/content/9/2/139.long)

47. http://thehealthinitiative.org/wp-

content/uploads/2012/03/Smokers-Timeline.jpg

48. https://www.braintumour.ca/Userfiles/documents/R
    esearch/CCRA%20Annual_2009_EN.pdf
49. http://www.tpsgc-pwgsc.gc.ca/bve-oae/rapports-
    reports/2008-609/index-eng.html
50. Source: Miller, N.Z. 2009. Vaccines: Are They Really
    Safe and Effective?New Atlantean Press, Santa Fe,
    New Mexico. p56
51. http://pediatrics.aappublications.org/content/119/1/
    222/F1.expansion.html
52. http://www.statcan.gc.ca/pub/89-628-x/2007002/c-
    g/4183071-eng.htm
53. http://www.statcan.gc.ca/daily-
    quotidien/131203/dq131203a-eng.htm
54. http://commons.wikimedia.org/wiki/File:Total_healt
    h_expenditure_per_capita,_US_Dollars_PPP_%28alt
    %29.png

Made in the USA
Middletown, DE
11 April 2015